AUTHOR'S NOTE

High-quality, patient-focused medical care has been central to my practice and professional life. For almost 25 years, I've been a primary care physician. I'm board certified in both Internal Medicine and Pediatrics. At Ellis Medicine, the health care system where I work, I see patients, as well as serve as the Medical Director for Primary Care. I've chaired the Pharmacy and Therapeutics Committee and presently chair the Quality Oversight Committee that oversees quality for the entire organization. I'm also a member of the Ellis Medicine Board Quality Committee and the Ellis Medicine Provider Quality Committee. Finally, I'm on the board of our physician's group, Ellis Medical Group, and chair their quality committee. My active involvement in the medical community has all added to my enjoyment of medicine and my passion to make it better.

My career commitment to better healthcare and my personal vision of what our healthcare system can achieve with teamwork and a little effort are what motivated me to write this book. I hope you enjoy reading it as much as I enjoyed writing it.

CONTENTS

INTRODUCTION: TRAINING CAMP

IN MY 20-plus year career as a primary care physician, I've constantly thought about the best way to deliver top-quality healthcare. Primary care physicians are often the first line of care for patients, and my job revolves around being an advocate for their needs. I recommend specialists when more intensive and specialized care is needed, and sometimes I consult with other doctors regarding an individual's medical history and condition.

But medicine has become more complex in recent years. The medical profession has always required extraordinary training, energy, and commitment from individual practitioners, but the system itself has become more complicated with increasingly convoluted procedural requirements on everything from insurance claims and billing, to prescriptions and specialist care. Along the way, the patient got lost in the shuffle.

While the system may be getting more complex, what comprises quality care is simple and can be boiled down to three core components:

- Competent physicians and other healthcare professionals;
- The quality of information and resources shared and communicated; and
- More engaged patients who work hand-in-hand with their doctors and providers.

More than ever, I've come to the conclusion that quality medicine requires a new way of looking at patient care.

Getting Everyone into the Game

I'm a fan of professional football. Like many sports, football is a game that depends on how well the coach and the players on the team work together on and off the field. During game time, the team works together to execute on plays, which are preset strategies and drills that every team member knows by heart.

Now, imagine a football game where the coach signals a play to the quarterback, calling for a 20-yard pass down the sideline. These are very specific instructions that the coaches decide to call based on a variety of factors—from their gut instincts and professional expertise, to observations on what's happening on the field and the performance and defensive stance of the opposing team.

Now, what if the receiver decided, on his own, to cut across the middle instead? If you've ever watched a football game, you know the disastrous consequences that can ensue with a botched play, and the colorful conversation that the coach will have with his players afterwards that are replayed and discussed on ESPN. A better outcome, of course, might have occurred if everyone on the team had followed the original plan, or at least communicated their concerns to the coaches on changing tactics beforehand.

Why Teamwork Matters in Patient Care

Over the years, I've found myself telling my patients and their families that medicine is a team sport and that *everyone* needs to get into the game and play. Physicians are familiar with this concept and know how to coordinate with their staff and other practitioners, but they often find it difficult to work with their patients. Patients and their families are an integral part of the game, and yet they are often passive or absent players. All too often, they see themselves as mere *recipients* of care rather than participants.

I see this type of disconnect between doctors and patients in medicine every day, leading to situations as mild as having to do multiple visits and administering treatments that aren't necessarily appropriate, to situations as disastrous as life-threatening drug interactions. The best way to avoid these "game fumbles" is for patients to become players—more active participants in their own healthcare. This takes communication, planning, and follow-through. The more cohesive, prepared and organized the medical team is—of which patients are an integral part—the better the results will be for everyone.

Why is it in your best interest to join the team? Two big reasons: getting quality care and reducing costs. These are often complex and intertwined with each other.

Get Better Quality Healthcare

The majority of Americans today have more than one medical problem. According to a 2004 report from the Center for Disease Control and Prevention, *Health United States 2004*, five out of six people age 65 or older took at least one medication and half of them took at least three medications. Many Americans will experience several chronic health problems, including heart disease, diabetes, and cancers. According to the World Health Organization, many of these diseases can be prevented or the chances of developing them significantly reduced.

How? With better teamwork between doctors and patients, I believe that people can buck these trends and lead longer, healthier lives. Good teamwork will get you the preventive testing you need, better evaluations for your medical problems, and the least amount of medication necessary to manage health conditions and get the job done.

Drive Down Healthcare Costs

Another reason encouraging patient involvement is more important than ever is that it will markedly reduce healthcare costs. For years, healthcare costs have been increasing at alarming rates. In 2008 dollars, per capita spending (i.e. money spent on each person) in the U.S. was the highest among 18 developing countries. We spent $7,538 compared to Switzerland's $4,647, Germany's $3,737, and Japan's $2,729.[1] And even though we spend the most money of any country in the world, we don't have the best health outcomes. What are we getting for our money? A study comparing the U.S. with Australia, Canada, Germany, Netherlands, the U.K., and New Zealand showed that we weren't performing all that well for the amount of money we spend. We were 4th in effective care, 6th in quality, 7th in safety, and 4th in patient-centered care.[2] In 2011, for infant mortality we were 41 out of 45 developed countries.

To do better and enhance our performance on a cost-basis, it's crucial that doctors, medical staff, and especially patients know how to play. As baby boomers retire and the population in the U.S. gets older, hospitals, insurance companies, and taxpayers will be bearing the brunt of increasing medical bills and healthcare costs. In this country, since January 1, 2011, 10,000 people are turning 65 years of age daily. By

---

[1] Organization for Economic Co-operation and Development (OECD), April 2011, http://www.oecd.org/health/healthataglance (accessed May 30, 2012).

[2] Karen Davis, Ph.D. et al., Common Wealth Fund, June 23, 2010.

2030, one in five Americans will be 65 years old or older. We need to control our costs or future generations will end up footing the bill.

How to Use this Book

While there is increasing awareness that to get the best possible care patients need to become more pro-active with their own healthcare, the conversations I've had with hundreds of patients over the years have shown that many people *still* don't know how to get into the game.

The goal of *Medicine is a Team Sport* is to get patients into the game by teaching people what they need to know to become more engaged in their own healthcare. This book won't turn you into a doctor. I'm not asking you to become an expert on every disease you encounter and to know all your treatment options by heart. There are numerous resources available out there to provide that information.

Rather, I want this book to be the guide that shows you how to join the team for the most important game in your life—your health. As a physician, I can tell you that doctors and other healthcare providers are the most invested when patients are interested and committed to their own care—and provide better care as a result. By getting involved, not only can patients increase their own personal satisfaction, they can improve their own health outcomes, too.

Sports have always been about the spirit of teamwork and collaboration—and that's precisely what drives medicine, too. *Medicine is a Team Sport* is divided into nine core chapters. Each chapter uses a particular sports analogy to illustrate important healthcare principles, which I hope makes the material more accessible and easy to understand. Here's what you'll learn as you go through the book:

1. **The Huddle:** Find out how to communicate and share important healthcare information with your team members, including your physicians and family members.
2. **Calling the Signals:** Maximize a visit to the doctor's office and convey the right type of information for an effective and accurate diagnosis. Avoid calling the wrong play with self-diagnosis.
3. **Understanding the Play:** Understand what key questions patients should be asking their doctors and strive for clarity on all plays.
4. **Special Teams:** Identify and work with other healthcare professionals that come into play to support your healthcare.
5. **The Playbook:** Learn how to manage special healthcare events and conditions, dubbed "game changers," that patients may encounter throughout their lifetimes and how to deal with them through teamwork and communication.
6. **Changing Players - Trades and Drafts:** Master the rules on how to switch physicians and to find the right physician for your needs when things don't work out.

7. **Situations to Avoid:** Dodge the common mistakes that patients make about elder care and proxy care.
8. **Equipment:** Discover popular monitoring tools and devices.
9. **Coaches Corner:** Hear the words of advice directed at other healthcare providers and family members.As you read each chapter, an overview of the topics is presented followed by examples and cases from my practice to illustrate what and what not to do as a patient. Sections conclude with a "Coach's Rx" that details my personal recommendations on what to do to become a better player and practical, actionable advice and tips to get you into the game.

Are you ready? Let's play.

ONE:
THE HUDDLE

IN SPORTS, the huddle is a gathering of team members to discuss strategy. In the Introduction, I talked about three components critical to quality care: doctors and other healthcare practitioners, information and resources, and patients. The intersection of these three elements takes place in the "huddle."

Who are the key players in your huddle? In your huddle, you're joined by all the doctors who take care of you, as well as by the medical staff involved in your care on the field. In the medical huddle, information—one of the three components we discussed—is exchanged.

Communicating with Your Team

Good communication is an absolute cornerstone in quality healthcare. If you're seeing more than one doctor, make sure that your medical record is shared with everyone. All your doctors should review your medical history, as well as know all the medications you have been prescribed and any other critical notes about allergies, recent surgeries, and pre-existing conditions. You may think that some of this may feel like overkill, but you would be surprised to know that details are often missed in the tangle of multiple visits with different physicians. More often than not, these "missed" details can have critical relevance for your care.

Case in point: If you see your eye doctor, you may think that your ophthalmology records don't need to be shared with your primary care physician or other specialists. I have an elderly asthmatic patient with glaucoma who was on an inhaler containing a steroid for her asthma. One of the side effects of steroids is a risk of potential increased vascular pressure in the eyes. My patient was deathly afraid of losing her vision. So, without informing any of her doctors, she stopped taking the asthma medication.

In the months she had ceased using her medication, she soon developed shortness of breath as her asthma worsened. At her next visit with me, we discussed possible reasons why her breathing had deteriorated. We talked about her other ailments, and I found out she had recently been to the eye doctor about her glaucoma. After digging further, the truth finally came out. She told me what she had done and how she had changed her regimen.

As her doctor, I knew I needed to get her in the game.

So, we called a "play." I advised her to return to the asthma medication, as the risks with inhaled steroids are lower than the risks with the oral steroids. A copy of my notes with my concerns and recommended plan of action was shared with her ophthalmologist, and we all coordinated. During her subsequent eye check-up, she had her ocular pressure checked to see if she was having any adverse reaction.

Shortly after that visit to the eye doctor, I asked her to come in to see me so that we could re-evaluate her overall health risks and see whether or not we would keep her on her asthma medication, or if I needed to find her alternatives. Her ocular pressure was normal, she reported, and it appeared there was no risk to her vision from taking the asthma medication. In fact, her breathing had improved and her energy levels had increased. Her asthma symptoms were under control. She felt great.

This "huddle" of all of us working together, coordinating and planning ahead, led to a better and healthier outcome for my patient.

Coach's Rx:

- **Share all medications and treatments prescribed by other doctors.** Medications that are prescribed for one condition may affect other systems in your body. Make sure your doctors know what medications and treatment recommendations are being implemented outside of their individual encounters with you. If you're seeing a new specialist or other healthcare provider, make sure you inform your primary care doctor. By doing so, your doctor can ask the right questions and make sure conflicting treatments are avoided.

- **Share all critical information with all partners and encourage communication.** If you have a doctor who isn't in the communication loop, get him or her in the huddle as soon as possible. Sometimes, you may have a few members who fumble on this. As a teammate, let them know that critical information exchange is a priority for you. Generally, your healthcare providers will respond positively and are happy to coordinate with others if you ask. If someone continues to fumble, consider "making a trade" (discussed in more detail in Chapter 6)—finding a new doctor that values communication and respects the "huddle" the way you do.

- **Don't be passive when communicating with your doctor.** When you meet with your doctors in your huddle, here's what I recommend: Make sure everyone knows the full reason why you're there. Provide a background history on key medical conditions. At minimum your doctor expects to hear about your symptoms, but there are often underlying causes that go unheeded because of lack of communication (more on this in Chapter 2).

  Many times, the problem with doctor visits is that patients view the experience as a passive one. They visit the doctor to get advice and often feel little compulsion to share. Or, they may feel their physician "knows best" and leave it up to them to deliberate on the best course of action. The problem is that passive deference can often lead to a partial and imperfect view of the situation. Your doctor can only take appropriate action when all the facts are on the table.

- **Trust your doctor.** The best way to reach desirable outcomes for all parties in the huddle is to make sure you raise your expectations of your physicians' role and your own role in interactions. Trust and respect go hand-in-hand with a willingness to share information and listen to what your doctors recommend.

TWO: CALLING THE SIGNALS

WE ALL know that one of the important aspects of communication in the "huddle" is talking to your doctor and relaying the right information. In football, players have 30 seconds to start a play. Likewise, when patients are at the doctor's office, they only have a certain amount of time to spend with their physician. Unfortunately, you aren't the only patient that needs to be seen that day. Managing the limited time you have with your doctor means having the opportunity to share your complaints and voice your concerns about a particular ailment. In addition, your doctor wants to do a good evaluation and offer a clear explanation that addresses your concerns and answers your questions. All of this needs to be done well in the allotted time.

Your team is now lined up and ready to run a play. You, as the quarterback at this stage, step up to "call the signals." What does this mean?

Just like in sports, your signals should be specific, clear, and understood by everyone. The ball is hiked: You're now playing to win this game as a team. Efficient doctor visits—knowing how to call the signals—is the lesson in this chapter.

Getting the Most Out of Your Doctor Visit: Focus and Preparation

The visit to the doctor's office is often the only opportunity you have to voice a particular complaint or seek advice about your health concerns. Make it count by calling the right signals. Primary care physicians, for example, only have about an average of 15 minutes to spend with each patient. During a visit, expect your doctor to:

- Ask you a series of questions;
- Perform a physical examination;
- Determine a diagnosis; and
- Prescribe the necessary treatments.
- Fifteen minutes isn't a lot of time, so patients and doctors together have to make the encounter really count. The fix? Focus and preparation: For each visit to the doctor, ***focus*** on just one or two of the most pressing concerns (in Chapter 5, we'll discuss the importance of follow-up visits), and be ***prepared*** to share descriptive, specific details about those concerns—the "signals"—with your doctor.

Focus: Prioritize What You Share

Patients are often tempted to bring a list of complaints on visits. These are often ailments or health issues that have been going on for a while, often for months. Some patients, knowing they have an appointment coming up, decide to wait and accumulate all of their concerns. It can be tough for your doctor to diagnose one or two ailments, let alone a slew of concerns shared on a single visit. With the average visit clocking in at 15 minutes or less, there just isn't enough time. In an effort to beat the clock, patients and doctors end up rushing the conversation, which can lead to mistakes and misdiagnoses. By limiting your conversation to a few complaints and concerns, you keep the visit focused, and your doctor is more likely to give you the best diagnosis. I'll talk more on what to do if you have a long list of concerns in the section on doctor visits in Chapter 5.

Prepare: What to Tell Your Doctor

Doctors want to know specific details about your condition or concerns during your visit. The following are guidelines of what doctors find useful to know about your condition during a visit. The list may look simple, but many patients have a hard time being descriptive in just the right way about their condition. So, here's what we look for:

- **WHAT has been bothering you?** List all symptoms that you have been experiencing, such as pain, nausea, digestive problems, fever, confusion, or respiratory issues. Let your doctor know where it hurts and how the pain feels. Be as descriptive as possible. For example: *"The pain is sharp and throbbing on my left side in between my ribs"* or *"I've experienced diarrhea and vomiting, accompanied by a fever of 102 degrees on two occasions, and I've noticed that my left temple throbs."* Indicate if anything makes the condition better or worse.

- **WHEN have the symptoms started?** Timing, onset, and frequency are important characteristics of your symptoms that help your doctor assess how serious or chronic an ailment or injury is. Your responses here will help shape the way doctors think about the problem. Give specific details about when problems started, when they appear, and if they are chronic or occasional. For example, don't just tell your doctor you've been having pains "for awhile"—for some people this might be a few days, while for others it could mean a few months. Instead, break it down like this: "*I've been experiencing these headaches for a week now (timing). It started right after I got back from my usual 10-mile run (onset) and I've been experiencing them every time I do any form of aerobic exercise (frequency).*"

- **HOW LONG do these symptoms last?** Along with timing, duration also lets your doctor determine a proper diagnosis. For example, a low-grade headache that lasts for several hours in the morning can signal a very different health problem than a sharp, debilitating one that induces vomiting, but only lasts a few minutes at a time throughout the day.

Intensity, timing, onset, frequency, and duration of your symptoms are all “signals” that your doctor “reads” in order to make a professional diagnosis. Preparing ahead of time the details of what is going on not only helps you focus on your body, zeroing in on what is really bothering you, but also paints a detailed picture for your doctor to help produce an accurate diagnosis.

Remember, your doctor isn’t a mind reader. And with the 15 minutes he or she has to see you, many things can be inadvertently overlooked because of lack of communication. This idea may seem rather obvious, but you’d be surprised at how many people underestimate its importance. Patients clam up or offer murky details about what they are feeling. Sometimes, they leave out important context clues, such as old injuries or circumstances that might illuminate the onset of an ailment. Trust me: The answers and information you volunteer shape the way your doctor thinks.

Be Cautious About Self-Diagnosis

Increased transparency and accessibility of medical information on the web has been a boon, but also a bane, to patient care. While patients are more educated about their health, easy access to information has also led to the problem of misdirected self-diagnoses.

Over the years, I've seen more and more patients who are keen on diagnosing their own ailments. Armed with information they gleaned from Web M.D. and other similar websites, they rattle off a series of "theories" of why they feel the way they do. Or, they become over confident about a particular course of action they should take and they look to me for affirmation, rather than my expert opinion.

While I support this enthusiasm among patients to take their health into their own hands, especially those who are prompted to live healthier lifestyles as a result of educating themselves, I also want to offer some caution: Over-zealous self-diagnoses can often do more harm than good.

Case in point: I had a patient who suffered from a couple of urine infections. One day, he found himself in the emergency room (ER) with severe back pain. He had experienced back pain with a previous urine infection, so his family simply assumed that a urine infection was the cause, and, with certainty, told the ER physician. The man was treated for a urine infection, and then sent home.

Later, when I saw him in my office, he told me the treatment wasn't working, and the back pain had continued unabated. The family was again adamant he was experiencing another urine infection. Strange, I thought. I looked at his labs and came to a startling conclusion: He didn't have an infection after all. In fact, I ultimately diagnosed that he had suffered a spontaneous fracture in his spine. This facture—not a urine infection—was the underlying cause of his back pain. It's difficult to predict what would have happened in the ER if his family had simply described his symptoms, and it might have saved him a few days of agony.

Coach's Rx:

- **Saying "I don't know" is OK.** Please, don't feel embarrassed if you don't know the answer to a question from your doctor (more details about clarifying doctor advice is discussed in Chapter 3). Too often, people tell me information to a question I didn't ask, and I have to ask again until I get what I need. Any confusion and back-and-forth between you and your doctor can be reduced if you simply stop and say, "I'm not sure what you're asking me. Can you explain that again?"

- **Express your concerns and opinions after you've given your doctor the necessary information.** Feel free to offer your opinion to your doctor, but do it in a way that contributes to the process. If you have a thought or information from another source that may shed light on your condition, then present them to the physician in the form of question, such as, *"Could diagnosis X be a consideration?"*

For example, if you think you might have pneumonia, first describe your symptoms. Then, ask your provider to consider the possibility. Your doctor may then ask you a few more questions to support or rule out this diagnosis. But whatever you do, let your doctor make the final call. If you're still unsure about what your doctor advises and recommends, ask questions. Remember, you and your doctor are on the same team and everyone involved is equally invested in winning the game.

- **Don't rely heavily on self-diagnosis.** The role of the patient is to tell the doctor what is wrong. In turn, the doctor's role is to figure out why. Frequently, patients misinterpret their own symptoms. They do a few hours of research online or hear about an experience that a friend had, and they immediately jump to some conclusion. While I welcome the empowerment that comes with self-driven research, I highly recommend against using the information you gather as a substitute for your doctor's opinion. From my own experience, extraneous information often sets doctors on edge and deliberately biases an interpretation and diagnosis. Well-intentioned but pushy patients can inadvertently derail their visit by prompting their doctor in the wrong direction. If you do have a concern about a particular diagnosis, mention it to your doctor in the form of a question for him or her to sort out.

THREE: UNDERSTANDING THE PLAY

IN SPORTS, players refer to their strategies out on the field or on the court as "plays." In medicine, a play might be a diagnosis and a plan of action your doctor recommends to help you get better. From prescribed medications and recommended regimens, to tests and specialist visits, "plays" can vary. To win the game—that is, getting better and leading a healthier life—everyone on the team has to have the same understanding of all the plays called; that is, everyone should know the game plan.

Throughout my 20-plus years of practicing medicine, it wasn't uncommon to hear patients complain that a physician didn't explain things or share important information with them. While I'm sure at times this is true, the vast majority of doctors do try to explain things to patients. The problem is making sure the message comes across in a clear way. As doctors, we like to think we explain things plainly. Unfortunately, patients and their families don't always tell us if they didn't understand something. Sometimes, patients might not even know they misunderstood. They simply accept their doctor's words at face value and nod in agreement. Without sharing their true feelings, their doctors are, in turn, oblivious that something might be misconstrued or misinterpreted.

Asking Questions

Not only should patients be comprehensive about the reason for their visit (see Chapter 2 for how to describe symptoms or conditions), they should also ask questions.

After hearing you describe the intensity, timing, and duration of your symptoms, your doctor may follow-up with other questions, do an examination, and then give a diagnosis. As your doctor gives his or her opinion on what might be happening and recommends certain treatments or tests, *make sure you understand exactly what's required of you*. You won't be able to play the game if you don't understand the plays your doctor calls.

Case in point: I have a lovely elderly patient who has aging kidneys. As I explained to her the details of her condition, and what she should expect in terms of treatment, I looked to see if she understood. I thought I had given a clear explanation and expected us to wrap-up the appointment. Instead, she looked at me with a smile and said, "Give me the third grade explanation."

We both laughed, and I was relieved. We regrouped, and I simplified my explanation. She was engaged in the conversation, stopping me when she needed a point clarified. At the end, she repeated back to me the main points, assuring me she had gotten it. Remember, we can only play well together if you, the patient, contribute on the field by asking questions.

A second case in point: A patient I had sent to

gastrointestinal specialists came in for a visit for other issues. During her visit with me, she recounted to me how she was told by a specialist that she had refused a test. She considered herself a good patient, so she wasn't quite sure how to come to terms with the actions she took. I asked her what she had told them when the specialists had suggested the test. She told them "No," she explained.

As difficult as it was for her to accept, I told her that she had refused. Coming to terms with the fact that she was also responsible in the decision process with her doctors was hard to stomach. As we talked, I found out that she had refused the test because she simply didn't think the specialists would find anything. After we discussed the impact on her health a bit more, she finally agreed it would be in her best interest to undergo testing.

In cases like this, patients often decline to undergo treatments or medical tests because they don't understand the procedures and what consequences on their health and well-being refusing could have. I told her, as I tell my other patients, "Ask questions if you're unclear or worried about a procedure." In her case, the specialists probably explained the tests, but something got lost in the communication process. A few questions on her part probably would have quelled her worries.

Finally, a third case: A patient came in with her daughter for a check-up. As I detailed the plan and answered their questions, I noticed the daughter writing down notes on a pad of paper. I caught this out of the corner of my eye and smiled. The patient said, "I want to remember everything." Taking notes is a great idea at doctor visits, and I encourage patients to write down their doctor's instructions and recommendations to avoid any confusion or misunderstanding later.

In your typical football game, players in different positions are expected to perform certain tasks: You have the quarterback, the linemen, and the running back, for example, all doing their part for the team. As a player in your own healthcare, you, too, have a responsibility at your position to perform certain tasks. This means understanding what needs to be done and knowing the role you need to play.

Coach's Rx:

- **Ask questions if you aren't sure.** In my own practice, I encourage my patients to ask me questions if they aren't sure about something. Don't just blindly give responses to questions that weren't asked. I've had patients who were unsure how to respond and volunteered information I didn't ask for to deflect from the fact that they were confused about something I said. This is unhelpful. The most important take-away is this: Don't nod your head and say you understand if you don't. You may feel deferential toward your doctor and be quick to accept everything explained to you at face value, but it does a disservice to your team and especially to yourself if you walk out of the office with the wrong game plan.

- **Confirm your understanding.** Summarize the game plan or plays back to your doctor before you leave the office. If you can't, then tell the doctor which part you didn't get and have him or her explain again. Don't feel embarrassed to ask for clarification. As you should now know, we're all on the same team and everyone is equally invested in winning the game.

FOUR: SPECIAL TEAMS

IN MEDICINE as in sports, there are particular situations that require special teams to take charge of your care. Special teams come into the game at certain times depending on your needs. In fact, these teams aren't involved in every play and may only be on the field a few times during the entire game. But even if they aren't in the game on a regular basis, special teams are crucial.

Let's talk about a couple of special teams you may encounter over your lifetime. These are mostly institutions other than hospitals involved in patient care:

- Nursing homes and assisted living facilities;
- Nurse home-visits (Visiting Nurse Association); and
- Hospices.

Nursing Homes and Assisted Living

Because of the specialized care and facilities they provide, nursing homes and assisted living facilities are often the best alternatives for elderly patients and seniors, as well as for patients that need round-the-clock care. These facilities come into play for patients who aren't healthy enough to be active participants in their own healthcare and medical needs. In most, if not all cases, the burden of responsibility usually falls outside the resident's hands, with staff, doctors, and family members playing a greater role.

How do they play a greater role? Many nursing homes today offer "subacute rehabilitation," which is an arrangement that provides recovery care for patients after or in place of hospitalization. Patients receiving this type of therapy are often elderly or debilitated, or those recovering from an acute illness and require extra time to recuperate before being fully released. For those who don't need to extend their hospital stay, but cannot return home just yet, nursing homes provide the space and care for extended convalescence. Subacute rehabilitation can take several weeks to a couple of months depending on the patient's condition.

Assisted living facilities provide a home for people who can't live on their own. The care provided is less intensive than at a nursing home, and residents can often do things for themselves. Unlike nursing homes, assisted living facilities have limited nursing staff and personnel. Usually, an assisted living resident goes to his or her own doctor or sometimes the facility will have a staff doctor on hand who manages the care of the residents.

Whether patients are staying at a nursing home or at an assisted living facility, they need to learn who is on their team and designate the necessary roles. As a good player in this situation, inform your teammates how you want to be involved and that you would like regular and timely updates. Communicate with family members and your providers your personal preferences for your care. If possible, decide on whether "proxy care" (see Chapter 7) is something that needs to be arranged in advance.

Case in point: I have a patient with mild to moderate dementia living in an assisted living facility. She experienced significant weight loss due to poor food intake. I ordered some supplements and the facility has been very good with providing these. When she and her daughter come for visits, her daughter reports back to me with details on her mother's eating habits. All members of the team—myself, my patient's daughter and the assisted living facility—have been successful in working together, communicating, and sharing information that ensures that the patient gets the best care.

And here's a story from personal experience on how communication with special teams is vital: My mother, who is in a nursing home, was admitted to the hospital because of wheezing and respiratory distress. Nine or ten months prior to this, her diet in the nursing home had been changed from solid foods to pureed foods because she had experienced difficulty swallowing. When she was admitted, the hospital received the information about her pureed diet, but didn't get the reason for the change. I stepped in to provide this information to the physicians in the hospital, which helped her medical evaluation.

Visiting Nurse Association (VNA)

Another special team to have on your side is the Visiting Nurse Association (vnaa.org). Sometimes when patients are released to return home after a stay at the hospital, they may still need extra care that only a healthcare provider can offer. For example, if you're recovering from major surgery, or are undergoing therapy after a stroke, a visiting nurse can be indispensable in providing hands-on care when you need it in your own home. Also, if you're taking care of another family member, a visiting nurse provides the extra support—getting you organized and keeping you and your loved ones in the game.

Let's look at this example: I had a patient who was a diabetic and had an underactive thyroid. Both of these conditions were not well controlled. When she came into the office with her daughter, we all talked about the changes that needed to be made. The new game plan was complicated: We needed to add more medication for her diabetes and adjust her thyroid medication. For a diabetic patient with a thyroid condition, these changes require precise and timely doses. Errors or deviations can be life-threatening. In a hospital setting, nurses would be on hand to organize a schedule and administer the drug, but my patient lived at home. She didn't have a regular caregiver at the time except for her daughter who stepped in on occasion to help.

Shortly after this visit, my patient suffered a stroke and

was admitted to another hospital. When she was discharged, she went to live with her daughter while she recovered. I had given her daughter a copy of the medications she was using. We later discovered that her mother hadn't been taking the medications as prescribed. After a long discussion, we decided we needed to bring in a special team: the VNA.

With the help of a visiting nurse, her daughter learned to administer her mother's medication on her own, and we returned to my patient's original medication regimen. Because of the special team, we were able to increase the quality and level of care for her mother. The end result was that my patient brought her diabetes and thyroid condition under control without having to change the medication or dosage.

Hospice

A hospice specializes in end-of-life care for terminally-ill patients who generally have six months or less to live. We often think of hospices when we think of cancer patients, but many hospices today also work with patients in the final stage of other diseases, such as heart or lung failure, and other serious conditions. Hospices have their own nurses and physicians on staff to provide this type of specialized care. These organizations serve a special purpose: providing comfort and compassionate care to the seriously-ill and helping people in their last days to die with dignity. Hospices help families understand what is going on during these times of crises, giving support and easing the transition. I don't think you'll regret having them on your team if that ever becomes necessary. Over the years, I've had multiple patients and their families using hospices and all have found the experience a positive one.

Coach's Rx:

What makes special teams work is how well information is communicated among all members of the team. In the beginning of this chapter, I mentioned that patients often play a limited role on special teams. However, I believe patients can still do their part when special teams are called on to the field during a game.

- **Keep your primary care physician in the loop.** If you're admitted to one of these special facilities, request that your primary care physician or the hospital share your medical history and records. Check to see what is transmitted; sometimes the information may be scant or provides very little background information to the special team. Your best bet in this situation is to take a more active role (or have a designated family member take an active role) in sharing your medical information. Any information that you supply to the staff physician will be invaluable.

- **Share all critical information with your special teams.** Sharing information ensures seamless continuity in your medical care. This is especially true for patients that move from one institution to another or receive care from multiple providers. A hospital or facility may only know the patient for a very brief time. Making sure information about past medical history and events are shared ensures that your special team calls the right plays and helps you win the game.

FIVE:
THE PLAYBOOK

IN OUR lifetime, we may experience life and health events that require close coordination with a physician or other healthcare provider. As we go through our 20s, 30s, 40s, and then middle age, retirement, and beyond, our medical needs naturally change. In general, the type and frequency of doctor visits depend on our age, health, and well-being, which in turn determine our susceptibility to a number of chronic diseases and health conditions.

In this chapter, we'll focus on some of those events—the "game changers"— that you're likely face in your lifetime, specifically:

- Infant development;
- Diabetes;
- Hospitalization;
- Cancer;
- Playing the internet doctor; and
- Doctor visits.

Some of these game changers concern joyful experiences (e.g., infant care and child development for parents), while others are more serious and emotionally trying situations (specifically, hospitalization, diabetes, and cancer). The last two—playing internet doctor and doctor visits—are more commonplace, but warrant a spot in your playbook, too.

That list isn't meant to be an exhaustive one. What I want to do is focus on the conditions or events for which patients don't usually see the immediate value of a more collaborative approach. In my experience, people faced with these particular game changers often call plays alone or break from the huddle too soon. Communication breaks down. Patients and their families don't coordinate with their doctors. To tackle these game changers and call good plays, it takes teamwork and close coordination among you, your doctor, and family members.

Keeping a Health Journal - Your Personalized Play Book

Before I get into our playbook, let's talk first about building your own personalized one. I highly recommend that you keep your own personal playbook in the form of a health journal. Why? A health journal lets you keep track of important health issues you encounter, helping you spot trends for certain health problems, and to gauge your overall health and well-being. Keeping all of this information is also instrumental for you and your doctor. Here are several ways a personal playbook can help you at the doctor's office, particularly when tackling game changers:

- **Personalized record of health problems and procedures:** Use the journal as an ongoing record of the health problems you've had and procedures that you've undergone in the past. This is particularly useful if you travel and if you ever end up in the emergency room, for instance. Medical records may not always be accessible, especially if you're traveling overseas or when internet connectivity is down. Having a record on hand is also a great way for you to review your medical history with your doctor to make sure you're both on the same page during visits.

- **Travel assurance:** Think of a health journal as a more personalized and mobile form of your medical record. For those who travel frequently, a journal can give you the peace of mind if you ever have to visit a hospital or see a doctor that doesn't have access to your medical records. Having all the necessary information at your fingertips that you can easily share with a doctor at different locations is a lifesaver.

- **Tracking medications and dosages:** In your journal, keep track of your medications, including dosages and the number of times per day you need to take each one. In addition, keeping a duplicate of this information on a small note card in your wallet is extremely convenient. I encourage all of my patients to do this. Previously, I used to give out medication cards, which patients could keep in their wallets for easy reference. But paper cards are being phased out as we move toward establishing electronic records. While going digital can be convenient in some respects, it also has its downsides—what do you do if the connectivity goes down, the computer crashes, the files become corrupted, or the power goes out? By keeping information about your medications in a physical location like a journal or note card, you can access the information anytime, anywhere without being dependent on an internet or network connection, or power source.

- **Reporting symptoms:** Before a visit, check your journal and make note of any observations that might help in a diagnosis. Seemingly unrelated symptoms may actually have significance; a record helps you keep track of these details. I have patients who keep journals, and we have found it tremendously useful when we need to access information about an experience or procedure undertaken over the years or since our last meeting.

If you have the extra time and want to be more diligent in keeping track of your health at home, here are other ways your journal can help:

- **Diet and exercise:** Keep track of diet and exercise habits as part of an overall plan to lose weight or manage cholesterol levels or blood pressure.

- **Self-monitoring:** Determine the cause or triggers of chronic ailments, such as depression, allergies, headaches, or gastrointestinal problems. In all of these cases, a journal can help patients keep track of when symptoms strike.

- **Mindfulness:** Beyond being a record of information, the act of journaling itself can have some psychological benefits. It teaches you to listen to your body and to be mindful of your thoughts and feelings, which can do wonders in reducing stress and helping you feel more in control.

Infant Development

Infant development is a popular topic of conversation among families and their doctors. Nothing is more game changing than the arrival of a newborn. Virtually all parents have similar questions and concerns as to the normal development and care of their children. Parents are naturally anxious that they are doing everything right to raise their children, watching out for immunizations, diet, and sleep and growth patterns. So, how can parents work with their doctors and keep being good stewards for their children's health and development?

During check-ups, the doctor is looking at three areas of

development in your child to determine normal growth and health: (1) Motor or physical activity; (2) socialization, or how a child reacts to his or her environment; and (3) communication ability.

At each stage of development from birth and throughout infancy, your doctor will check for "milestones,' or expected actions or behaviors, exhibited by your child. For example, at two months of age, infants can be expected to lie on their stomach and lift up their chest with their arms. At two months, parents should note their children bobbing their head a little bit. They will also respond to an adult voice and smile. Doctors look for these relevant milestones to determine how well your child is progressing and if there are grounds for concern. Numerous books, such as *Caring for Your Baby and Young Child* (Bantam Press), contain solid information for mothers, fathers, and caregivers from the American Academy of Pediatrics on specific milestones.

Before any parents out there become overly concerned and anxious that their children aren't meeting particular milestones, remember that every child is unique and develops and matures at different rates. Milestones only serve as general guidelines. Even children from the same family may exhibit different patterns of development. While we expect children to hit certain milestones at certain ages, not every child does so uniformly. So the question becomes: When should parents be concerned?

Delays in development milestones are NOT necessarily signs that something is wrong with your child. However, if there are developmental issues in more than one area, or if a developmental issue in one area persists, then this may be cause for concern.

Case in point: I recently did an exam on a one-year old. He walked very well, pointed, was social, and ate well. He said "mama" and "dada"—but not with purpose; in other words, he wasn't speaking the words to the appropriate parent. However, the rest of the exam was normal, and I told the parents we would continue to watch him over the next few months. My advice to parents who observe irregularities like this is not to panic. While I took note of these minor communication issues, I'm pretty sure his verbal skills will mature and "catch up" by the time I see him again at the next doctor visit. In those first few years, some children just grow and change in their own time.

Coach's Rx:

Your doctor will work with you to determine the best course of action for your infant or child. Here are several actions you can take to ensure the accuracy of a diagnosis:

- **Track your baby's development in your health journal** (see the previous section in this chapter). If you observe delays in any of the three critical areas of development—motor activity, socialization, or communication—take note of them.

- **Let your doctor know about any genetic diseases or health issues in your family.** Is there a history of autism or other developmental concerns? Talk to your family members and ask them to share whether they experienced a developmental delay in their own children and to identify what the patterns were. Then, share this information with your doctor. Often, the delays may just be isolated events. In time, the baby catches up.

- **Track any development delays.** If a delay persists over several months or over several areas, consult your doctor. Together, your team will create a new game plan to address these issues.

Diabetes

Many experts agree that there is an epidemic of diabetes in America. Not only are adults affected, but also children and teens are experiencing escalating incidences of diabetes. In fact, you probably know several people in your family or among your colleagues or friends who have this disease. By far, it is one of the most pervasive health game changers that doctors and patients will face.

According to the American Diabetes Association, nearly 26 million children and adults in the United States—around 8% of the population—have diabetes.[3] In 2007, the total cost of the condition, from direct medical

---

[3] American Diabetes Association, "Data from the 2011 National Diabetes Fact Sheet," http://www.diabetes.org/diabetes-basics/diabetes-statistics/?loc=DropDownDB-stats (accessed April 30, 2012).

expenses to the costs of work loss, disability, and premature mobility, is estimated to be $174 billion. Diabetes also causes more deaths every year than breast cancer and AIDS combined, and two-thirds of people with diabetes suffer a fatal heart attack or stroke.[4] Risks factors for diabetes include being overweight or obese. Family history, ethnicity, and age also play a role. In fact, many people assume that eating habits and weight are the only risk factors that matter. But many overweight people never develop diabetes, and many people with diabetes are at a normal weight or only moderately overweight.

---

[4] American Diabetes Association, "Diabetes Myths," http://www.diabetes.org/diabetes-basics/diabetes-myths/ (accessed April 30, 2012).

What is Diabetes?

Diabetes is a metabolic imbalance where the body is unable to produce enough insulin to process sugars in the blood stream to be used as a source of energy for our bodies. Insulin is a hormone released by our pancreas that moves the glucose, the sugar in our blood that we get when we digest food, into the cells in our body. The entire process, regulated by insulin, transforms food into energy.

When you have diabetes, your blood has elevated amounts of sugar because: (1) Your body can't produce the right amount of insulin to break down the sugars and get them into your cells; and/or (2) your cells aren't responding properly to the insulin produced. As a result, glucose builds up in the blood, and you don't get enough energy.

This sugar buildup can have dire consequences. The biggest concern is that the sugar imbalance in the blood creates an internal environment in the body that can damage organs and adversely impact other bodily systems. In fact, if diabetes isn't controlled well, it can lead to serious debilitating issues, such as heart attacks, kidney disease, damage to internal organs, and in extreme cases, amputations of affected limbs and even premature death.

While medical research has produced breakthroughs in treatments for patients suffering from diabetes, there is no known cure. The best play to call when you face diabetes is prevention.

Prediabetes and Prevention

The number one way to treat diabetes is through prevention. Before one even reaches the threshold to be called a diabetic, there is a condition called prediabetes, where your blood glucose levels are higher than normal. What sets prediabetes apart from diabetes is that it can be handled without the use of medication if diagnosed early. To determine if you have prediabetes, your doctor measures your fasting blood sugar.

Unfortunately, prediabetes usually doesn't elicit as much concern among patients because it isn't yet full-blown "diabetes." Over time, however, prediabetes can also damage your body if not treated—just like diabetes. I urge people to take their prediabetic conditions seriously. Without taking any action, those with prediabetes have about a 30% chance of developing diabetes. I can't tell you how many times I have seen this occur over just a few years in patients who ignored advice and didn't take preventative action.

Coach's Rx:

- **Be prepared to follow a strict regimen and make lifestyle changes.** Depending on your condition, your doctor and/or diabetic educator will advise you on how to change the way you eat, recommend a weight loss program (notably, a positive impact on blood sugar levels can be observed after the loss of as little as five pounds), and/or prescribe medication to control your blood sugar. Because of the potential problems associated with prediabetes and diabetes, treatment criteria can be even more stringent for people who have other health conditions, such as high blood pressure or asthma, which compound the adverse effects.

- **Manage the medication and treatment.** Diabetics generally wind up having to take some form of medication or insulin treatment. A typical diabetic may be on 3-5 medications for diabetes-related high blood pressure and on 1-4 medications to manage the diabetes itself. Not only is keeping track of these pills difficult for some people, but it can also get very expensive.

What's the game plan to minimize the medication and treatment deluge?

- **Educate yourself.** Staying informed and knowledgeable about your condition and what you can do to help yourself is extremely important. If you're diagnosed with prediabetes or diabetes, your first course action is to educate yourself. *Knowledge is power.* Hospitals, treatment centers, and clinics all employ certified diabetic educators. Take advantage of these services. These professionals can teach you about your disease and what you can do to help manage your condition, such as dietary tips. Many people think this is silly and don't "want to go to class" or "do the homework." The truth is the more you learn about the disease, the more empowered you'll be in taking charge of your own health and well-being. Educating yourself about risk factors, treatments and medication gives you the opportunity to take control.

Choosing not to educate yourself is like trying to play football without knowing the rules. Armed with the facts, you can minimize your medication needs and, in some cases, treat the diabetes without taking extra medications for years. A few of my patients have made successful strides in this direction using this strategy.

- **Take advantage of preventative care programs.** If you're worried about the costs of seeing a diabetes health professional, talk to your health insurance company. Most likely they have similar programs to encourage you to take preventative action (or programs to help you keep your condition from getting worse). Most plans will pay for the classes and even compensate you for yearly updates and check-ups should you need a refresher. Many people don't know this and don't take advantage of it.

- Insurance companies are generally more than happy to pay for diabetes education, which decreases your chances of contracting a much more serious (and costly) condition, such as heart attack or stroke, as a result. Medicare is a leader here, covering initial diabetic education and up to two hours a year thereafter for refreshers as needed. How much money can be saved from education? Having a stent put in place because of a diabetes-induced heart attack can easily bring a hospital bill over $10,000. Compare that to preventative diabetic classes and consultations, which may cost a few hundred dollars. It really pays off.

- **Act now to prevent or halt complications.** Diabetes has an insidious effect on our entire body, damaging our kidneys, nervous system, eyes, and other organs. Make sure you listen to your doctor and get into a good diabetic program sooner rather than later.

Hospitalization

Hospitalization is a fast-paced game changer for many reasons: Conditions on the field (your health) can worsen or improve quickly; players (your doctors and nurses) may substitute often; and the business of medicine has changed. In the past, it was a much easier game. When you were admitted to a hospital, your family doctor took care of you. If a specialist was needed, your family doctor recommended one and the specialist paid you a visit and gave his or her input.

Today, things are different. Over the last ten years or so, hospitals have moved to a model of employing doctors called "hospitalists" who only work in the hospitals. Many primary care physicians don't work at hospitals anymore. Even the specialty doctors, such as cardiologists, work in large groups and may rotate around to different hospitals.

What does this mean for patients who are hospitalized? While in the past you may have seen the same set of doctors for your needs, today it's not uncommon to see a different set of doctors every day during your stay. A doctor may see you only for a day or two, and the partners in his or her group take turns filling in thereafter. A hospitalized patient may see anywhere from 2-7 doctors from various physician groups during the same hospital stay that may last less than a week.

Here's a typical scenario: You go to the emergency room (ER) Thursday night. You get admitted and see the admitting hospitalist. The next morning, you wake up and are seen by a new hospitalist; the other one has already gone home. On Saturday morning, there might be a new hospitalist for the weekend. Less than 48 hours in the hospital and you may have been seen by at least two or three hospitalists already. At the end of the weekend, there may be another new face. Other consulting groups that might be called in during your care will also have their own rotation of doctors who pay you a visit and may also change just as quickly.

Seeing so many doctors during a hospital stay also makes discharge more complicated than ever. When it's time to leave the hospital, patients sometimes make the mistake of thinking that they can let their guard down. But team effort still counts and here's why: Post-hospital care depends on a very important document called the "discharge summary." Discharge summaries detail specific instructions for continuing patient treatment at home or in a nursing home, if needed. Without that document, members of your team won't know what to do next. Discharge summaries require careful coordination with your team.

Case in point: I saw a patient after a hospitalization and had a copy of the discharge summary for his post-hospital care. The summary mentioned an out-patient test that was to be done. However, there was no mention in the discharge summary of *when* the test would be done. Should I order it? Did the hospitalist doctor or specialist order it? I didn't know. Fortunately, the patient's wife was on top of things and knew when the test would be scheduled.

Another example: I had a patient who had been home three days. When the patient came in to see me, no discharge summary was provided. While in the hospital, the patient had fluid taken out of an ankle, though this wasn't the main reason for the stay. I had no clue as to why this procedure was done; neither did the patient. While the patient was in my office, I called the discharging physician. He was somewhat embarrassed that he hadn't yet provided a discharge summary, but was able to give me the information I needed, so I could treat my patient. Without this information—which would have been listed on the summary if one had been completed—I was stuck.

With so many people involved when it comes to hospitalization, how do you call the right plays to win the game?

Coach's Rx:

- **Designate one family member as the point person on all communications with doctors.** It can get very complicated for doctors who may find themselves fielding a flurry of phone calls from spouses, siblings, or parents all asking the same questions about the patient. That is why families should designate a single point person who will be responsible for speaking to the doctors and disseminating information to the rest of the family.

- **Identify and get in touch with the admitting doctor.** When patients are admitted, it's the admitting doctor and his or her group that will be in charge of the patient's care, overseeing day-to-day visits and checkups, and making the final call for treatments. For example, if a patient goes through the ER, he or she might see several doctors, but the admitting doctor will be responsible for the patient's care. On communications about the hospitalization and care, the admitting doctor is the first point of contact for the designated point person.

- **Arrange to get frequent updates from the admitting doctor.** From day one, the point person should inform the admitting doctor that the family would like daily updates: the patient's condition, important tests to be ordered, and the plan for the next day or two. Ask the admitting doctor about the other doctors consulted on the case. Find out: (1) which doctors will be seeing the patient and be personally involved in the care, and (2) which days during the hospitalization will the doctors be seeing the patient. If there is a change in schedules, get the name of the new doctor who will be seeing the patient to avoid any surprises.

- **Ask the admitting doctor to coordinate with the patient's family doctor.** If the admitting doctor isn't the patient's family doctor, ask what the procedure is for contacting the family doctor for information. Making sure the patient's family doctor and the admitting doctor coordinate is absolutely essential. Many families neglect to do this and critical information can be missed. This is also an opportune time to make use of the patient's personal playbook (discussed earlier in this chapter).

- **Observe that quality care basics are enforced.** Make sure that whoever comes to see the patient has practiced basic hygiene 101: hand-washing on the way in and out. Hand-washing is the number one way to stave off life-threatening infections and complications but is often overlooked.

- **Make the point person reachable.** Reaching a physician, especially if you aren't the patient, can sometimes be difficult. Doctors are busy professionals with hectic schedules. They may not be on-site every day at the hospital where the patient is admitted. Always give the admitting doctor an accessible number, such as the point person's mobile phone number. This makes it easy for the doctor to call about updates and minimizes frustrating phone tag.

- **Double-check all medications prescribed.** One of the most important actions I can recommend for patients is reconciling all medications with the admitting doctor when being admitted and before being discharged from the hospital. Reconciling medications means defining what medications the patient is or will be taking. Unfortunately, medication reconciliation is one of the hardest things to do and can be riddled with inaccuracies despite the best intentions from patients and doctors. At times, the digitization of medical records has worsened inaccuracies. This is because many hospital electronic programs pull medication records from pharmacy databases. Since a database is downloaded unfiltered, the records are often riddled with obsolete data on patients, such as medications that are no longer being taken. This can be a challenge to sort out in the office during a visit with your doctor, and even harder to verify in the emergency room where doctors are unfamiliar with most patients they see.

These kinds of small errors can quickly build up and cause a chain reaction. For example, if the list obtained on admission is inaccurate, or if the database housing the patient's records contains a data glitch, the errors will carry through until the patient is discharged. Even if the list is correct on admission, the discharging provider may sometimes makes a mistake.

To minimize a snowball of errors, here's what I recommend: The patient or point person should keep a list of the patient's medications, including dosages and instructions on administering. On the day of admission, discharge, or in an office visit, the patient or point person should go through the list with their doctor, the discharge/admitting nurse, or provider. Make sure all of the medications taken at home prior to the office visit or hospitalization are accounted for in records, even if the patient is no longer taking them. I've seen patients come home on duplicated medications. Remember, if you're not sure, ask and confirm that you and everyone else have the right information on hand.

- **At the time of discharge, ask when the discharge summary will be done.** When it comes time for your discharge from the hospital, make sure a discharge summary is provided promptly. Some doctors are very good at doing them the day of discharge. However, others aren't—and this causes problems for your family doctor or other providers who may be taking over your care. Also, some discharge summaries are better than others. Ask your family doctor if a summary was written well. If not, make this known to the hospital so this can be corrected.

As we discussed in Chapter 3, information flow is vital to making sure everyone on your team, from your family members to your primary care physician, understands your medical needs. Focus on improving how you communicate with the doctors involved during a hospital stay. The plays you ultimately make during a hospitalization affect your life or the life of a loved one.

Cancer

Cancer. The very word elicits strong emotions and fear among most of us. Cancer is actually not one disease but a broad name for a group of more than 100 conditions. Cancers can ravage any part of our bodies and systems: There are bone cancers, ovarian cancer, breast cancer, skin cancer, and leukemia. This game changer's broad-based nature can be bewildering for patients. The emotionally-wrought experience of diagnosis and treatment can also lead patients and their families to fumble simple plays. The abundance of information online and misinformation about many types of cancers also prompts families to make misguided decisions.

What is Cancer?

Different types of cancer abound, but all cancers can be defined as abnormal cell growth in the body. Cancer cells are essentially healthy cells that grow out of control and invade healthy cells in the body. The causes of cancer are varied, but they are related to some form of damage to our DNA, which can be caused internally (inherited abnormal DNA) or induced by the environment (e.g. bad diet, smoking, or too much sun exposure). In normal cells, a damaged cell either repairs itself or dies. With cancer, the damage isn't repaired, and the cell continues to reproduce abnormal cells. If left untreated, cancers can cause serious illness and even death.

Diagnosing Cancer

While there are many types of cancer, there is a fairly common approach to dealing with all of them. During a check-up, your doctor may find an abnormal growth in your body. Usually this begins with the discovery that the body has a growth or a "mass" somewhere. At this stage, it's generally unclear what caused the growth and how serious it is. The fumble: *making assumptions about these initial findings.* Often, cell growths in the body turn out to be benign (non-cancerous) so your doctor will advise you that further tests are needed.

During my career, I have seen many instances where the discovered masses we thought were cancer were in fact benign. Until a biopsy is performed, which gives your doctor a more definitive look at the nature of the cell growth, don't make any assumptions. A similar sports rule that accurately describes the caution patients should heed when it comes to treating cancer: *Don't try to run before you have the ball.*

Case in point: I have a female patient who had suffered from lymphoma (a type of a blood cell cancer). She had received treatment, did well, but faced the possibility of recurrence. One day, she came to my office complaining of a new rash on most of her body. I was worried because I knew of a type of lymphoma called Sezary's Syndrome that exhibits an itchy rash similar to what she observed.

I wasn't sure what she had, but mentioned it as a

possibility. Because of her experience, she and her family had some familiarity with lymphomas. When I told her husband that Sezary's Syndrome could be one of the possibilities, he started asking me about treatments. I told him we were not there yet and emphasized that we still did not have the diagnosis. We needed further testing and I did a skin biopsy. My reassurances did little to quell his anxiety. The skin biopsy showed that the rash was psoriasis which resolved with the use of steroid creams.

Another example: A patient of mine found a mass near one of his kidneys. We all initially thought it had to be kidney cancer (we would have been right 9 out of 10 times). He went through an evaluation, which included a biopsy, and we waited. And waited. In fact, the diagnostic outcome changed four times before we could definitively confirm a correct diagnosis. With the use of sophisticated genetic tests, we were able to determine the exact diagnosis. Throughout the period of uncertainty, the family kept its spirits up and approached the evaluation process with patience. The patient and his family knew that treatment would depend on the right diagnosis, so they were willing to work with their oncologist and avoided jumping to conclusions.

For many people, the waiting and uncertainty during the cancer evaluation process can be agonizing. But testing requires your utmost patience and nerves of steel. Give your doctors time to make sure everything is done right. With the threat of cancer looming, emotions can run high, but be careful about letting your emotions dictate decisions because this can lead to unnecessary fumbles on the field. I know it's hard with a condition like cancer, but patience is a virtue.

After testing, if the diagnosis is indeed cancer, your doctor will move to the next play: gathering information about the disease to find out the extent of it and your prognosis for treatment and survival. In doctor's language, this is called "staging the disease." Generally, there are four stages: Stage 1 is a very local disease, and stages 2-4 mean that the cancer has spread to some degree. What stage cancer you have determines the treatment and care you receive, as well as your overall prognosis for survival.

Because cancer is complicated and induces a strong reaction in patients and their families, let's review our playbook.

Coach's Rx:

- **Keep a cool head and don't jump to conclusions.** Avoid making any assumptions. Work only with the definitive facts you have. Take one day at a time and work with your doctor. Cancer evokes strong emotional reactions, leading individuals to make hasty decisions before tests results come in, or rattling the nerves of families before all of the facts are available. An initial diagnosis of cancer is stressful, but try your best not to "jump offside" before the ball is hiked. Test results can offer good news, too, so listen to your doctor and wait. Even after biopsy results come back, the results may still be ambiguous and more detailed genetic tests may need to be done. Be patient: It will pay off.

- **Screen your research with your doctor.** One of the most common mistakes is getting too much information from doing research on the web and jumping to wild conclusions about the disease without first consulting your doctor. Without proper guidance, too much information about treatments and survival rates can skew or cloud your perception of the cancer. Reading that you do on the web or at your library is fine, but try holding off any intensive research campaigns until *after* you hear back from your doctor on a diagnosis and after the stage of the cancer has been determined. Then, coordinate with your doctor to review the information you find. Trying to manage the deluge of information you find on your own, many of which won't apply to your case, can be emotionally taxing, too. Save yourself the grief.

- **Get a second (or third) opinion if you wish—but only *after* work-ups have been done.** Many times, families want other opinions about a cancer diagnosis. After all, everyone wants the most accurate assessment and the best possible recommendations for treatment, and it's helpful to hear several medical opinions before making a decision about treatments and care. If the primary care doctor works near a medical school, which gives families access to different doctors, finding other physicians can seem like an easy option. However, I find that people move too quickly to find alternative opinions even before a comprehensive work-up is done. Rushing won't accomplish anything. Until the initial work-ups have been completed, you and your doctor are still in the dark, and it would be a waste of time and resources to seek out other opinions at this stage.

- **Resist the urge to go it alone.** Once you have some definitive tests, work with your primary care doctor to get recommendations on oncologists and experts to canvas. You don't have to do blind searches online or do it all on your own. One of the reasons patients try to do their own searches is because they worry they might insult their doctor by requesting a second opinion. Remember, we're all equally invested in ensuring the best outcome. Always work alongside your doctor; he or she will probably know someone with the right expertise who can help, and your doctor will often know these physicians personally. Play with your team and the game will be easier.

Playing the Internet Doctor

One time, a friend of mine recounted her success in treating a medical problem she and her husband were having. When I asked about her doctor visits, she shook her head. My friend had looked up the information she needed on the web. She joked that she was now an "internet doctor." (To her credit, she has some familiarity with the medical field and knew her limitations.)

While I applaud the access to information that the web has to offer, I also see several limitations and want to caution people. Uninformed online research can be a game changer—often with dire consequences. While my friend was able to find the information she needed and use it well, most people aren't as savvy. Here are two troubling situations I usually see: First, people experience symptoms and start doing their research online. Without much vetting, they gather all the information they scoured on the web doing a simple search on Google or Bing and present it to me during an office visit. Based on what they found, they then ask me how they should proceed. The problem with the information found this way is that there is often very little or no oversight over what gets published online. Often, the accuracy of the information cannot be guaranteed. As a result, people may find themselves sifting through a lot of junk information, which can do more harm than good.

Second, people jump to the wrong conclusions from the information they gather from a web search. Similar symptoms can manifest themselves for a wide-range of diseases and ailments. There are simply too many variables or scenarios to take into account when drawing a diagnosis. Unfortunately, I have seen patients treat themselves incorrectly or delay coming in because of false information they read online, or because they drew the wrong conclusions.

Here's an example: Recently, I saw a young teen suffering from prolonged headaches. She gave me an excellent history. I then did my evaluation and gave my opinion. But I also learned that she had gone online, researched headaches, and found distressing information on brain tumors. As her exam was normal, I talked about the fact that a brain tumor (a common concern) wasn't anywhere near the top of my list. The look of relief on her face was priceless. A few days later, we did a follow-up phone call, and the patient's mother reported her daughter was doing just fine.

Naturally, when people do an online search on headaches, the information that jumps out at them is usually related to brain tumors. What most people don't find online, however, is that brain tumors aren't pressing concerns on a doctor's pediatric checklist if the exam is normal. If the concern was brought up during the exam, I would have addressed it sooner and moved on.

Patients often tell me, "I bet you're going to hate this, but I went online and did some research on my own." I respond by saying, "Well, it depends on what you do with the information." We laugh, they tell me what they found on the web, and then we move on to address the issues.

Online research is just one of the many tools in your toolkit, but it's by no means an adequate replacement for your doctor's expert opinion. On the other hand, if done correctly, web research can sometimes pay big dividends. So, now let's talk about some good internet plays.

Coach's Rx:

- **When you see your doctor:** Make sure you describe your symptoms to your doctor in the right way (if you need a refresher, head back to Chapter 2). After you've told your physician your symptoms, describing in detail—the "What," "When" and "How"—then follow-up that you may have found a *potential* cause from your web research. Ask your doctor to share his or her opinion on your thoughts. At this point, you may be worried that you're overstepping your bounds. But if done in the right way, your doctor will appreciate your candor. Doctors love patients who show an active interest in their health.

  What is harmful is when patients insist on particular diagnosis based on what they read online without consulting their doctor's opinion. Keep an open mind and your doctor will, too. In this way, your doctor will work with you to address your concerns and confirm whether or not your findings are relevant.

- **After the diagnosis is made:** Doing web research in the right way can provide a wealth of information even *after* your doctor has given his diagnosis. For example, say, you're diagnosed with hypertension. You ask your doctor about diets that can lower your blood pressure. Your doctor may suggest looking up something like the "DASH diet." After this recommendation, you hop online to do some research and find recipes that meet the DASH diet criteria. Just don't forget to share your plans with your doctor. Showing that you're trying to help yourself and taking charge of your health not only motivates you but also your doctor.

- **Get recommendations to guide your online research.** Feel free to ask your doctor to recommend websites. A site that is vouched for by your doctor is always more reliable than one that isn't.

Doctor Visits

In Chapters 2 and 3, I went over in detail how to "call the signals" and understand plays, where we discussed best practices on how to get the most out of your doctor visits and appointments. In this section, let's discuss the doctor visit more strategically as a game changing play.

How do we run the doctor visit as a play? A popular recommendation for patients is to prepare before a visit by making a list of concerns to bring up. Lists can be very helpful tools. The problem is that lists can sometimes turn into lengthy ones that can be overwhelming and lead to a poor quality visit.

For example, for an appointment, your doctor may have expected to see you for your high blood pressure. However, you now want to tell him about that sore shoulder you've had for the last four months. You had an appointment so you waited to collect all your concerns and now want to share everything. Remember, you have only so much time with your doctor (usually 15 minutes), so you have to make the most of the appointment.

Let's look at the doctor visit from two different perspectives:

Patient's point of view: From your perspective, you want your doctor to look at your concerns, take each one of them carefully and thoughtfully, and have all your questions answered and treatment explanations given in a way you can understand. Fair enough.

Doctor's point of view: Doctors want to do achieve several things during a visit: (1) Assess the severity and nature of your problem(s); (2) manage them in the way you expect; and (3) keep their schedules on track to minimize the long waits in the waiting room of other patients like you. If a doctor has to listen to your long list of concerns, it detracts from time spent evaluating the more serious concerns you may have.

If doctors perceive that they won't be able to cover everything in the amount of time allotted for your appointment, there are several choices to be made: Doctors can either address your concerns, ignore them, or give your concerns minimal attention. Only the first scenario is ideal.

Here's an example: After finishing with a particular patient, I walked him down the hall and gave him his chart to bring out. Before I turned to leave, he asked me, "Doc, this chest pain I've been having is arthritis, isn't it?" I could have easily smiled, and said, "sure" and moved on to my next patient.

Instead, I said, "Actually, I don't know what this is. Come back tomorrow and see me." The patient did. With my full attention on this particular concern, we were able to delve deep into his symptoms. We discovered he was actually having angina, or pain in his heart, with exertion. If I had rushed to a decision in that previous appointment, either agreeing with him or ignoring his concerns altogether, we wouldn't have discovered the true nature of his condition.

Another example: Recently, at the end of a visit with a long-time patient, I was about to get up and conclude the appointment when out of the blue she pulled out a sheet of paper. She admitted that she had other concerns but was waiting until our consult ended to avoid interrupting me. I was a bit rattled, as most doctors would be at this kind of "ambush." I explained why this type of last-minute presentation is upsetting for doctors. We talked a little about her extra concerns and decided we would discuss them more at her next visit. At her follow-up, she presented her concerns up front—which turned it into a much better visit for the both of us.

So, how do you run a better play during your next doctor visit?

Coach's Rx:

- **Hold on to your list of concerns and focus on the pressing issues first.** When you sit down with your doctor, be up front that you have other concerns you would like to raise. List those concerns, and then ask which of them your doctor can tackle at this particular appointment. Depending on the complexity of your list, you may have to come back for a separate visit to address your other concerns in detail. Remember, a question you have may seem simple to you, but may be complex for your physician. Select the most important items, and let your doctor focus on those first. Come back to the others if necessary. In this way, you bring your doctor into the game in the best and most time-efficient way.

- **Make another appointment if necessary.** As we discussed in Chapter 2, going through a laundry list of complaints can be an inefficient way to handle your doctor visit. Sharing every single ailment won't produce a better diagnosis. With the limited time you have with your doctor, you may only be able to focus on a few specific conditions. Start with those most pressing problems first, and *be prepared to make another appointment*. Sometimes, for items we aren't able to cover fully, I can start an evaluation before my patient comes back. Not only is this incredibly satisfying for me, but also provides peace of mind to my patients. Remember, this is your health. Treat the time you have with your doctor with respect.

Suggesting another visit, if necessary, will instantly gain you respect and admiration from your doctor.

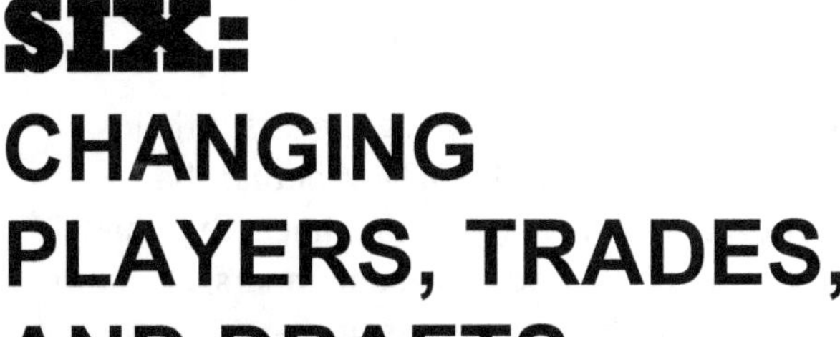

SIX: CHANGING PLAYERS, TRADES, AND DRAFTS

THROUGHOUT THIS book I've emphasized how the doctors and healthcare providers you work with are members of your team. But what if one or some members of your team just aren't working out? What if, after making all the right plays with your doctors, you still don't score—that is, get the care you're looking for?

Just like in sports, when players aren't performing well on the team or meeting expectations, you may need to draft new players or make a trade. As a patient, you have several options:

- You can put up with the current situation;
- If you're in a group practice, you can see a different doctor in the group; or
- You can leave the group and seek out a new group practice to find a new doctor.

If you're unhappy with your current doctor, I don't recommend simply tolerating the situation. After all, not everyone's personalities click and it's in your best interest to find a provider with whom you get along. But before you eject a player from the field, take stock of the situation and talk to your doctor first.

For example, many patients will gripe about their doctor to their friends and family. Whether the complaint is that a doctor talks too much, that the doctor doesn't have good bedside manners, or that the doctor rattled off the long names of prescribed medications without any explanation—more often than not the patient shares their concerns with everyone else except the person who might actually be able to help: *their doctor*. So, before you rush to change doctors, have a frank conversation with your provider and try getting some answers about your concerns. You may be surprised.

Case in point: I often give instruction sheets to patients to help them remember detailed routines on taking medication or undergoing treatments. One day, an elderly patient of mine came in accompanied by a relative. After the appointment, I did my usual routine and handed out the instruction sheet. During the follow-up a few days later, they complained that they couldn't figure out how to use the medicine I had prescribed. At that point, I was puzzled because the instruction sheet was supposed to help patients avoid a situation like this. I looked at the sheet I had given them and realized that I had accidentally given the wrong information.

I asked why they didn't call or let me know the instructions were unclear. They shrugged and said that they thought I looked upset during the last visit and were reluctant to ask for clarification. I don't remember being upset that day, and I was even more surprised that I gave off that impression. I promptly apologized for the confusion, but I learned a lesson that I always share with patients: *If your doctor's instructions look unclear to you, don't hesitate to ask for clarification.* It's their job to give you the best care they can—but they also need your input. Before you leave the doctor's office, make sure you clearly understand your doctor's instructions.

Coach's Rx:

- **Work it out with your physician first.** When you perceive a conflict, my recommendation is to first try and work out your concerns with your physician. This first step is the easiest because you already have a relationship with your doctor. The reality is that most doctors have a positive impression about their relationships with patients: They *think* they are personable, give good service, and offer clear advice. And doctors don't always know when they've fumbled the ball.

- **Use constructive criticism.** When you have decided to raise your concerns, do so in a nice and constructive way. Be honest but be constructive in framing your problems. Most physicians do want to make things right. Remember, we all have the same vested interest in winning the game with you, and we realize we can't do that without your trust.

- **If it's necessary, make the change *within* the physician group.** If the situation that makes you unhappy persists even after you have aired your concerns, then you have a choice: "making a trade." If you're with a practice with multiple physicians, try switching to a different provider in the same group. Sometimes personalities don't mix, and physicians recognize this, too. The trade doesn't have to be hostile. After all, your records are there and you may have good relationships with other workers in the practice.

- **Seek a new group and new physician—as a last resort.** If, even after making the trade, you still find yourself unhappy, it may be time for the final option: "going back to the draft" and recruiting a new physician. This is the hardest of your options for several reasons. Depending on where you live, you may not have a lot of choices. Physician practices may be full. Finding a new doctor is always hard. Many people ask their friends or family for advice. One can call the county medical society, too. Other people's opinions matter here, but take those personal recommendations with a grain of salt; you still have to do your homework and proper vetting.

- After you find someone, it's important to set up a "meet and greet" visit. This isn't for treatment, but just a meeting with a prospective doctor to chat and talk. Doctors are usually willing to do them. If I do them, I talk to prospective patients at the end of the day. At the meet and greet, discuss why you're seeking a change with a new doctor. This gives you a chance to see if you click with the new physician, and it gives the new doctor an idea of who you are and why you were dissatisfied. Any new player to your team will want to make the relationship work to get your team off to a good start.

SEVEN: SITUATIONS TO AVOID

IN THE game of life, there will be many instances that will ultimately cause undo stress to you and your family. I'm talking about special situations where patients become incapacitated in a way where they can no longer make sound decisions without the help of others. Let's go through two situations—elder care and proxy care—and how you and your family can make the best decisions to stop an emotionally trying experience from slipping into a full-blown crisis.

Elder Care

One of the most important demographic characteristics of the U.S. population is its rapid aging. Over the next few years, as more people retire, medical advancements become more mainstream, and our birth rate slows, a higher percentage of the population will be over the age of 65. As a result, elder care is becoming a pressing topic for many families. In fact, age-related diseases, such as dementia, are on the rise. According to researchers, the incidence of dementia in people over the age of 80 is almost 25% and increases dramatically in people over the age of 90.

What's challenging for many families is how to respond to a diagnosis like dementia. Many families delay taking action. The problem is that age-related diseases seem to strike family members at a time in our lives when we may be the busiest—with careers and our own kids, for example. With our busy lives, it's very easy to overlook or ignore the slow mental and physical decline of a parent who is suffering from dementia and living at home. Dementia strikes slowly and the symptoms are often manifested in ways that don't seem outwardly alarming at first. It can lull families into a false sense of security.

With dementia sufferers, what gradually happens is that they lose their ability to take care of themselves. As a result, before even life-threatening events take center stage, small things start to fall apart: bills may be missed, bank accounts left disorganized, and nutrition and health neglected from a lack of wanting to shop or prepare meals. It can then progress to being potentially very dangerous: forgetting to turn off the oven or faucets around the home, tripping or falling, or getting lost. Families seem to think that as long as the elderly relative isn't in "dire straits" they can look the other way. But this attitude can have serious consequences.

Here are several examples from my experience: For some families, dealing with a demented relative can be a relatively smooth experience. One patient of mine, a wonderful man, was fortunate enough to have strong family support. He lived with his wife who managed his care at home with the help of their children, several of whom were retired. The children took turns staying with their parents for prolonged periods of time to help. As a result, the man was lovingly cared for at home for 5-7 years where he peacefully passed away.

Not everyone is this fortunate. I treated an elderly couple where the wife suffered from dementia. Their children and children's spouses worked full-time and were unable to devote the intensive care and time needed for her care. They all did the best they could. As the wife's condition worsened, she got very combative. It was very difficult and embarrassing for her husband, who bore the burdens of her daily care.

A situation like this is one of the most difficult situations to treat medically, but is quite common. To make matters more complicated, the family was mired in the red tape of Medicaid enrollment, which significantly delayed the elderly woman getting into a nursing home. Despite their best efforts, the family's experience was emotionally shattering.

There are several actions you can take to avoid a crisis unfolding like that. Set up the right plays and learn them well to make the transition for your loved ones easier.

Coach's Rx:

- **Act swiftly at the first signs.** At the first sign of possible dementia, such as memory loss, confusion, forgetfulness, or changes in personality, make an appointment to see the doctor. It's in everyone's best interest to get your loved one evaluated as early as possible, and to start discussing future plans to provide support or alternate living arrangements before the condition worsens and becomes a crisis.

Unfortunately, what I see too often is that families bring their relatives to me when it's already too late; the patient is now so dysfunctional that living alone is no longer an option. Family members face a tough decision; many cannot just stop their lives to fix things. They feel scared, frustrated, and burnt out. They also assume that I can automatically get their ailing relative into a nursing home because I'm a doctor. The problem is that the system doesn't work that way, and doctors can't expedite the nursing home intake process.

Once a family member starts exhibiting symptoms, early action is critical to avoid the fumbles and bad plays that can quickly build up and burden families. Most of the things that need to be done have nothing to do with medical treatment, but with early action.

- **Explore your options.** Early intervention and planning matter. How fast the process works and what options are available to you depend largely on one's financial situation and the bed availability of desired facilities. If patients can pay for a space themselves, the process moves faster. However, most people can't. Look at your options early on: assisted living facilities, home health aids, or nursing homes. What can you afford financially in your area? Most of the difficulty is finding a facility one can afford financially and that family members agree on.

- **Steel your nerves, one yard at a time, for an emotionally taxing experience.** The decisions that need to be made about committing a loved one to a facility are never easy. Often, the involved patients are in denial that anything is wrong, and they don't want to leave their house or accept help. However, keep plugging away. In football, this is often referred to as "running plays up the middle of the field"—grinding out a few yards at a time. At some point, you'll break through for a big gain. If you've ever taken care of an adult who can't take care of himself or herself, you'll know it's a full-time job with overtime and no easy breaks. Don't get caught in this situation.

Proxy Care

Another situation to avoid is finding yourself in a position where your wishes aren't represented. This occurs most commonly when you, the patient, aren't able to speak for yourself. For example, you suffer a serious stroke or a mishap that leaves you in a coma. In situations like this, doctors consult family members about how aggressive or how much medical care *the patient would want if he or she could speak.* Family members have to make assumptions and make the final decision on your behalf. If no one is on your side, you may wind up having procedures done that you would not have wanted. You don't want people's emotions to affect the way you receive treatment. I've seen this happen and proxy care is the best way to ensure your preferences are heeded.

Coach's Rx:

- **Arrange for a healthcare proxy.** To avoid this situation where your life may fall in the hands of others, arrange for a healthcare proxy. This is a personal representative whom you pick in advance to speak for you and represent your healthcare needs. Once you have a proxy form filled out and notarized, bring a copy to your doctor and to the hospital. The proxy can then guide the staff to give the care that you would have wanted in situations where you're incapacitated.

- **For more serious and binding arrangements, fill out a POLST.** Beyond a healthcare proxy, there is also a POLST (Physician Order for Life Sustaining Treatment) program you can join, which makes more explicit what you want and don't want in terms of treatment. These exist in numerous states under different names. For example, in New York, it's called the MOLST (Medical Orders for Life Sustaining Treatment) form. POLST forms detail instructions for a wide-range of treatments, from administering CPR and using a ventilator, to whether to allow antibiotics, feeding tubes, IV fluids, comfort measures, and hospitalization.

- **Keep these forms up-to-date.** While the forms are binding they can always be revised to accommodate other wishes. If you update your arrangements, then inform your doctor and give him or her a copy of the necessary forms. Make sure the paperwork is in order to ensure that someone is always playing your position.

EIGHT: EQUIPMENT

LIKE IN any sport, knowing how to use the equipment is vital to how well you play the game. In this chapter, we'll review some of the common equipment that patients come across, from medication to monitoring devices, and go over how to use them properly.

Medication

In primary medicine, the equipment that dominates is medication. Patients handle this "football" in different ways. Some patients are like the wide receivers or running backs who love to get their hands on the ball: These types of patients want and take medications for everything. Others are like the linemen: They rarely touch the ball and when they do, they don't always know what to do with it; some of them don't ever want to touch the ball.

So, how do we handle the football? Let's look at two different types of medications in detail: nonprescription and prescription. We'll start with nonprescription medications.

OTC and Nonprescription Medication

Over-the-counter (OTC) medications may seem innocuous, and patients tend to abuse them or aren't mindful of the potential risks and side effects of taking them. Just because they are readily available doesn't mean that they are safer than prescription drugs. For example, people often don't pay attention to dosage recommendations. People may inadvertently give a dosage of cough medicine to a child that is really meant for an adult. In fact, there is a recommended ban by the Food and Drug Administration (FDA) on cold medications for children under the age of six based on studies showing that those medications may have dangerous side effects.

Take dextromethorphan, which is labeled on cough medicines as the "DM" at the end of a brand name (e.g., Robitussin DM). In an overdose, which can be easily happen in administering to small children, the medication can cause abdominal pain, increased heart rate and blood pressure, headaches, and agitation. DM can also be addicting and there is the risk of substance abuse.

Other examples of common OTC medication that can be easily abused are antihistamines. People use them for allergies, for which they work well—but they also use them for colds, for which they don't work so well. It's often easy to rely on antihistamines for colds because they seem to reduce the same symptoms (e.g., runny nose, sneezing, clogged sinuses) as those we experience with allergies.

What are the side effects? Take men with enlarged prostates. Men with this condition often have trouble urinating or their urinary stream is slower. One of the side effects of antihistamines can be a worsening of this condition, which can lead to urinary tract infections. This occurred with one of my patients. After a couple of urine infections, we figured out that they had occurred after he had a respiratory infection and had used antihistamines to treat it. Now that he knows the side effects, he no longer reaches for his allergy medications to treat the occasional cold and has never had another urinary tract infection.

Natural Supplements and Remedies

Natural supplements can also be problematic because the "all natural" description can lull people into a fall sense of security. Many people don't realize that natural supplements are also drugs, too. Unfortunately, while governing bodies like the FDA monitor OTC drugs, they don't regulate the health claims and medicinal properties of natural supplements.

Some of the most popular supplements that people buy over the counter from health food or alternative medicine stores are fish oil and Gingko Biloba. What many people don't know is that these supplements can have adverse interactions with certain drugs, such as a medication called Coumadin, a drug for inhibiting clotting often prescribed for people who have had blood clots or have an irregular heart rhythm called Atrial Fibrillation.

For supplements, we still don't know definitively what works and what doesn't. While some have become popular, such as fish oil for lowering the risk of heart disease, there are numerous other types of supplements for which science is still unsure. Most people read the labeling and take it at face value. But supplement claims don't have to be tested under rigorous conditions and subjected to clinical trials that prescription medications undergo. When studies are done, many supplements simply don't make the grade.

Many patients think the "medical establishment" is unfairly biased against natural supplements. But let me reassure patients that no big conspiracy by the establishment exists, nor is a cabal of medical professionals trying to prop up "Big Pharma." In fact, doctors often view prescribed drugs as "more work" because patients taking them must be checked for pre-existing conditions and monitored and tested for potential side effects. Doctors also have to watch for potential drug interactions if their patients are on other prescription medications. It's in the best interest of both doctors and patients to reduce the number of medications prescribed to the minimum needed to treat a health condition.

What does appeal to doctors is the integrity and transparency of information available. The three things we want to know about ANY medication, from OTC drugs to supplements, are: *(1) Does it work? (2) What are the side effects? (3) And how much does it cost?*

Unfortunately, with many supplements, we only really know the answer to the third question. If you look at the fine print on the packaging for supplements, you'll see that it usually says, "This product is not intended to cure, diagnose, treat, or prevent any illness" or "These statements are not approved by the Food and Drug Administration." So, if you plan to take supplements, especially if you're on other medications, practice caution and make sure your doctor knows.

Prescription Drugs

What about prescription drugs? We have all heard the term "over-medicated" and anyone who watches TV has seen the overwhelming marketing push by pharmaceutical companies to market their drugs. It's easy to feel a bit annoyed and overwhelmed by the apparent availability of a medication to treat every ailment we have, from sleeping problems to arthritis.

Many people fall into two camps: Some think that medications are the root of all evil, while others think they are wonderful. Whether you love or hate them, prescription medications have been instrumental in keeping people alive and in fighting some of our toughest diseases.

One problem I see with prescription drugs is that people can become overly reliant on them to treat their ailments. Medications become a substitute for direct action. In fact, some medications perform so well that people forget that they even have a stake in their own health. One type of drug that has become commonplace are statins (e.g. Lipitor), which are used to control and manage high cholesterol levels. These pills have been so successful in lowering cholesterol levels that people often neglect their diet or shun exercise, relying on the drug to do all the work.

One time, I tested the cholesterol levels of a patient who was on a statin. The test was not optimal, and she said to me, "I guess I *do* have to pay attention to what I am eating." She was right. If you don't do your part, the benefits of the medications you take can become diluted or even canceled out. Your doctor may then have to increase the dosage, which can lead to... side effects.

Side Effects

Side effects are the potential downsides to all types of medication people take and they can vary based on the type of medication, the dosage, and individual sensitivity. Sometimes we don't discover side effects until a drug has been on the market for a few years.

The media is fond of sensationalizing side effects that are discovered for popular medications. Unfortunately, it can often unduly scare people off medications completely. I have had patients stop taking their medications outright because of a story they heard on the news. The problem isn't that these patients are trying to be cautious, but that they forget to consult their doctors. Many medications, for example blood pressure and antidepressant medications, should not be stopped immediately.

Make sure you *always consult your doctor* when it comes to making a decision about your medication—

whether you want to change the dosage, frequency, or to stop outright. Your doctor will take the big picture into account and try to minimize the dosage (and thus the side effects) and number of medications you take within the limits of what's best for your overall health.

Case in point: Statins, used to lower cholesterol, can cause muscle pain in the form of some general achiness. My experience with statins and this muscle ache side effect is that when I have patients stop their medication, they usually start to improve in just a few days. If they don't see abatement in muscle pain, then we can rule out the side effect possibility and look for other underlying causes. By working with me, my patients and I can narrow down the possible causes of the side effect and determine the best course of action.

Unfortunately, I've had many patients who took themselves off their statins for months without informing me. This is a bad play. When I ask if stopping the medication helped, they say no, but they stayed off the medication anyway.

The fumble: making haphazard changes without consulting your doctor. If you feel you're having a medication problem, let your doctor know right away before making adjustments. Remember to work with your teammates before calling an independent play.

Oxygen

Oxygen is often misunderstood as a critical piece of equipment. That's right, I said it: oxygen. We all take it for granted. But there are those who need a higher grade than the 21% concentration we all breathe from the air around us every day. Unfortunately most patients don't like to use it. However, the reality is—for those who need it—oxygen is a lifesaving drug.

The most common example of how oxygen can save lives is in smokers who have a lung condition called COPD (Chronic Obstructive Pulmonary Disease). Doctors usually give these patients anywhere from one to several inhaled medications to treat the COPD. The medications don't prolong life—they just make patients feel better and some may help prevent hospitalization. The only things that prolong life for those suffering from COPD are: (1) stopping smoking, (2) lung reduction surgery for those who qualify, and (3) oxygen. If you need oxygen, not using is tantamount to choking yourself. Smokers and COPD sufferers have compromised lungs and without the extra help from concentrated oxygen treatments, simply breathing can put extra strain on the heart and other organs in their body.

Many people who are prescribed concentrated oxygen imagine bulky tanks being wheeled around. Those days are gone. The nice thing is that technology advancements have reduced the size of those tanks. Tanks are no longer the metal monstrosities that even spectators sitting in the nosebleed seats could see. Yes, those tanks still exist, but most people now have access to smaller, more portable tanks that are lighter and easier to carry. Remember, oxygen can save the lives of people who need it.

Monitoring Equipment

There are several pieces of equipment that help physicians and medical staff monitor your progress, including glucometers, insulin pens, needles, and blood pressure monitors. Let's go through each one.

Glucometers

Glucometers are blood sugar monitors often used for people who have diabetes. These monitors allow you to measure sugar levels in your blood. By checking sugars at different times of the day, you and your doctor can better plan your treatment. These monitors can also alert you to spikes in blood sugar that may be a symptom of something more serious. For example, let's say your sugars throughout the day are less then 150 on average and you see them start to rise. This can be an indicator that an infection may be starting. Of course, there are also other reasons sugars can increase; your doctor will work with you to analyze your glucometer readings.

A large variety of meters are on the market and most of them are easy to use. They come in different sizes, even devices so small you could carry them around in your pocket or purse. There are some with larger screens for easy reading, and some that need just the smallest amount of blood to do a reading.

Another significant advancement is in the ability to test your blood sugar in places other than your poor, aching fingers. If your diabetes is stable, you can test on the hand and forearm for example.

I've tried some of the new glucometers available on the market; the experience isn't bad at all. Work with your assigned diabetic educator and your doctor to find the right monitor that will suit your needs.

Insulin Pens

Another very important piece of equipment for diabetics are insulin pens. Many diabetics find it difficult and stressful getting their regular doses of insulin because of the hassle of administering injections and because of their natural fear of needles. The reality is that if you're a diabetic, you may be required to give yourself regular doses of insulin. As an alternative to conventional needles, insulin pens are a wonderfully convenient delivery system.

They offer two big advantages: (1) The insulin pens are idiot-proof. The companies that manufacture them have done a great job in crafting and designing them so that they are extremely easy to use. If your vision is an issue, many pens offer numbering labels that are easy to see. If you don't hear well, when you turn the dial of a pen, you can feel and count the clicks to get an accurate dosage. (2) The insulin pens actually do look like pens, which means they are extremely portable and can fit in your pocket. No more messy and embarrassing kits to carry around.

Needles

Frankly, most patients fear the dreaded needle, and it can be a downright phobia for many people. Maybe it reminds us of immunizations when we were kids when the needles used were intimidating and large.

Today, needles are so small—smaller than even the tiniest sewing needles—you almost need glasses to see them. Patients are amazed when I show them the size of the needles I use. Needles used for insulin injection are actually smaller than the needles you use to prick your finger to check your sugar. These newer needles also hurt much less or not at all. When patients finally experience a prick, they find the experience was more tolerable than they thought.

Blood Pressure Monitors

For people with hypertension, a blood pressure monitor allows them to monitor themselves, which is generally a good idea. The big issue is when there is a discrepancy between readings at home and readings in the doctor's office. Readings can naturally vary based on the type of monitor and the consistency of the medication regimen the patient is on, but it's still a good idea to check the accuracy of your monitors on a regular basis.

How do we handle that kind of situation? I ask patients to bring their blood pressure monitor cuff with them. While our readings won't necessarily match, they should be relatively close, say within 10 points. Doing this, I've had all kinds of results. Patients have had to get new cuffs because the readings were so wildly varied. Conversely, we've had good matches where the accuracy of the reading was actually better than on the office monitors. Once you buy a monitor, bring it with you to your next doctor visit, and have your physician check it against the office monitor.

How do you find the best monitor and cuff for your needs? That can be a little more difficult to answer. Sometimes, trial-and-error works best. Check *Consumer Reports* for product reviews of blood pressure equipment. And how about digital monitors? Digital monitors are becoming more and more accurate, with some even able to detect irregular heart rhythms. This feature can be important for you if you have Atrial Fibrillation, for example. A regular, non-digital monitor can't give as accurate a blood pressure reading for those who suffer from Atrial Fibrillation because it often misses the irregular heartbeats. In general, however, the cuffs that you pump up manually and listen to through a stethoscope are the best, though they can be very difficult to use on your own. Be sure to discuss your concerns with your doctor if you need help deciding which equipment to buy.

NINE: COACHES CORNER

IN MEDICINE'S dynamic environment, finding and paying for quality can be difficult, so the help of others is more vital than ever. Unfortunately, many patients overlook the extra help and resources that are out there. Remember, the more we all approach healthcare and patient well-being as a team sport, the more successful we'll all be in meeting our healthcare goals.

This chapter is directed at other players in the game that also contribute to patient care. Doctors are just one part of a patient's team. Other healthcare providers and supporters, such as dieticians, nurses, and health aides, as well as family members, can also serve as healthcare "coaches," providing patients with the necessary support and motivation.

Whether patients use these coaches to supplement the care they receive from their physicians, patients can turn to them for extra help and guidance beyond the hospital, clinic, or doctor's office.

Coaches, get in the game with patients. It will certainly make your job a lot more fun and satisfying. Now, go out and win one for the team.

Coach-to-Coach Rx:

- **Enlist the help of the patient's family members.** Family members can provide the extra ears and eyes in making the crucial observations to save a patient's life. For example, family members can sound out alarms about certain risk factors that the patients themselves might not have shared, such as that a loved one is a "fall" risk, has a habit of sneaking around cigarettes, or has shown an allergic reaction to certain foods or medications. This ensures that everyone has a complete picture of the patient and can take action to prevent any future problems.

- **Enlist the help of other healthcare providers and professionals.** To successfully treat chronic diseases, such as diabetes, many patients can benefit from the help of ancillary staff or organizations, such as diabetic educators, dieticians, and support groups. Invite these coaches to consult with you and provide your patients the extra care they need.

POSTGAME: THE LOCKER ROOM

IT'S been a long day. We've talked about a lot of things, from calling signals to potentially having to make a trade. We looked at some common plays, and while this certainly isn't an all-inclusive list, it gets us started on how to better play and win the most important game of your life—your health.

I'm always scouting for good ideas. If you have a story about working better with your team, share it with us at **Medicine Is a Team Sport** (medicineisateamsport.com). The website also features extra tips and strategies that have helped my patients and me over the years.

When it comes to your health, I believe that with the right plays and strategies we can all play and win the game.

Dean Limeri, M.D.

Head Coach, *Medicine is a Team Sport*

www.ingramcontent.com/pod-product-compliance
Lightning Source LLC
Chambersburg PA
CBHW051341170526
45166CB00002B/904